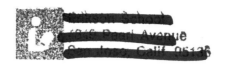

HANDS

HUMAN BODY

Robert James

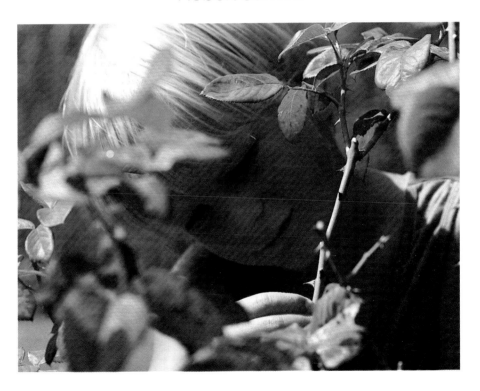

The Rourke Press, Inc.
Vero Beach, Florida 32964

PHOTO CREDITS
All photos © Kyle Carter except cover © Frank Balthis

Library of Congress Cataloging-in-Publication Data

James, Robert, 1942-
    Hands / by Robert James.
        p. cm. — (Human body)
    Includes index.
    Summary: Describes the anatomy of the human hand, how it dif-
fers from the "hands" and "paws" of animals, and its susceptibility
to injury.
    ISBN 1-57103-105-7
    1. Hand—Anatomy—Juvenile literature.   [1. Hand.]
I. Title II. Series: James, Robert, 1942- Human body
QM548.J36   1995
611'.97—dc20
                                            95–19037
                                                 CIP
                                                  AC

Printed in the USA

TABLE OF CONTENTS

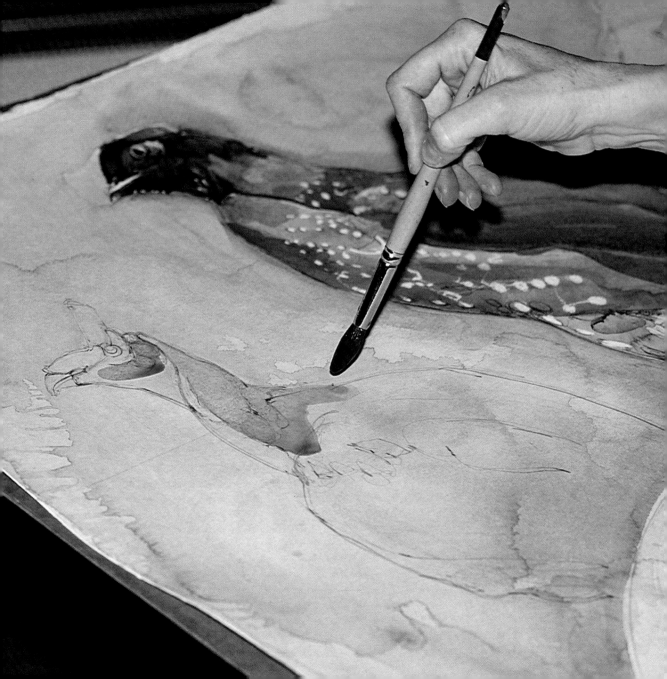

HANDS

Think about what separates humans from most other animals. Be sure to put hands at the top of your list!

Hands can do many wonderful things. Hands play pianos, grasp baseball bats, weave rugs, draw pictures, and punch computer keys.

Hands have many other useful purposes, too, in work and play. Of course, hands can also get us into trouble, like the hand in the cookie jar.

The hand of this artist paints
in water colors

USING HANDS

Hands are great grabbers and graspers. The fingers and thumb of a hand are designed to hold objects and pick them up.

Because fingers are so **flexible** (FLEHX uh bul), they do an amazing number of jobs for us. They work for us, scratch our itches, and even help protect us.

The thumb helps the other fingers by clamping against them. Try holding a juicy cheeseburger or shaking hands with just four fingers.

The fingers and thumb make a great grasping team

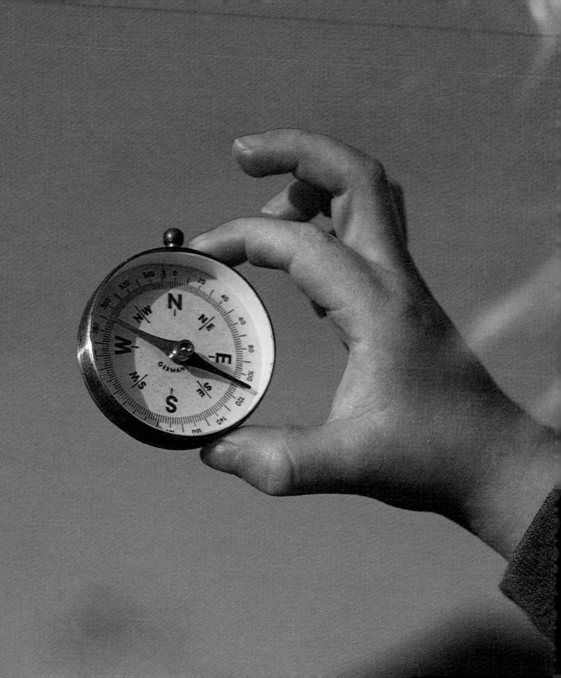

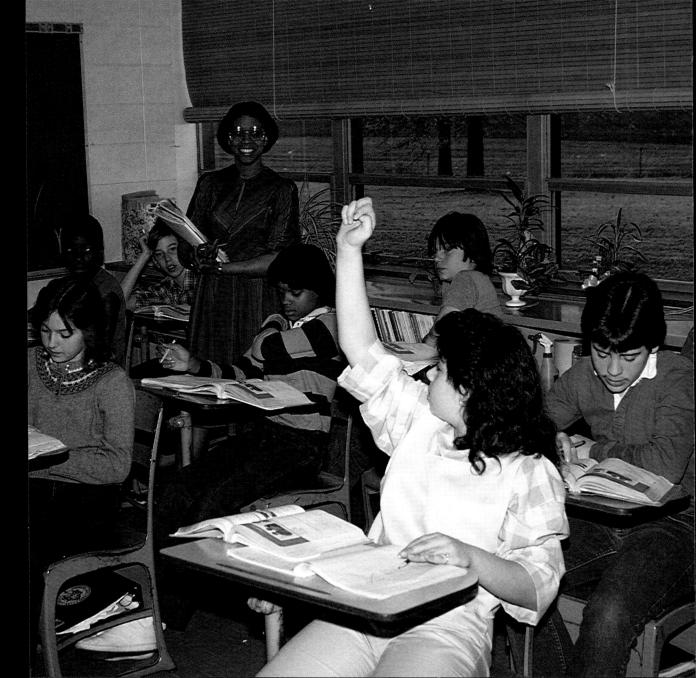

TALKING WITH HANDS

People often use their hands to help make themselves understood. A choir director waves in time with the music. Deaf people communicate through hundreds of hand signs.

People's hand signs are **gestures** (JEST yurz), or signals. Common hand gestures may mean peace, victory, goodbye, come here, number one, success, or—with thumbs down—failure.

People without sight learn to read with their hands. They feel the letters of the **Braille** (BRAY el) alphabet with their fingers.

A raised hand in a school class carries an unspoken message

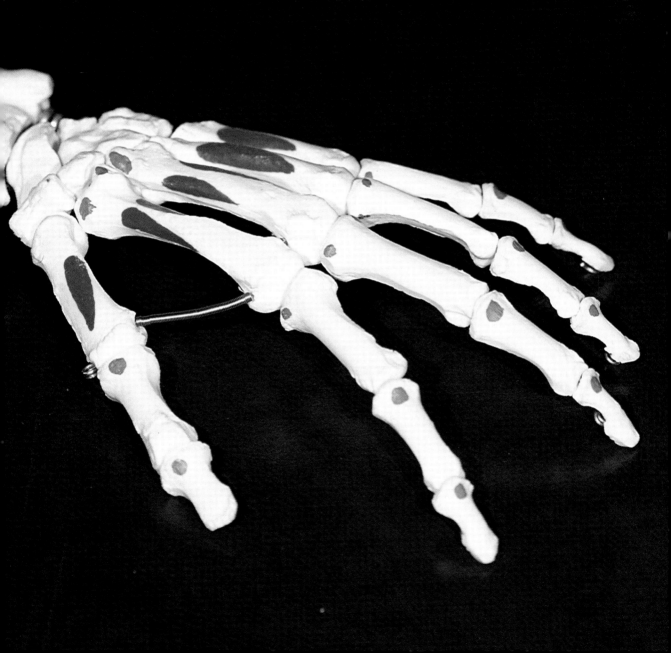

PARTS OF THE HAND

The hand begins at the wrist, the foremost part of the arm. The underside of the hand is the padded palm.

Inside the hand are muscles, tendons, ligaments, blood vessels, nerves, fat, and 27 bones.

The flesh that makes up the muscles, tendons and ligaments moves the hand.

This model of a hand shows the bone structure

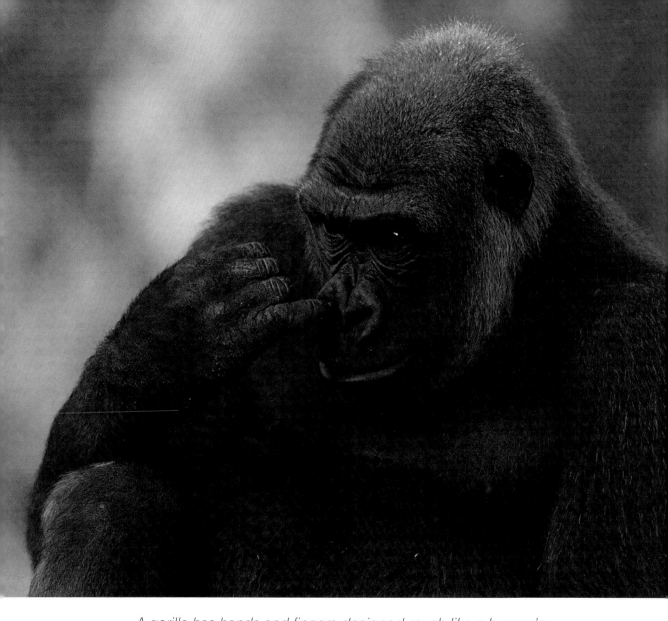

A gorilla has hands and fingers designed much like a human's

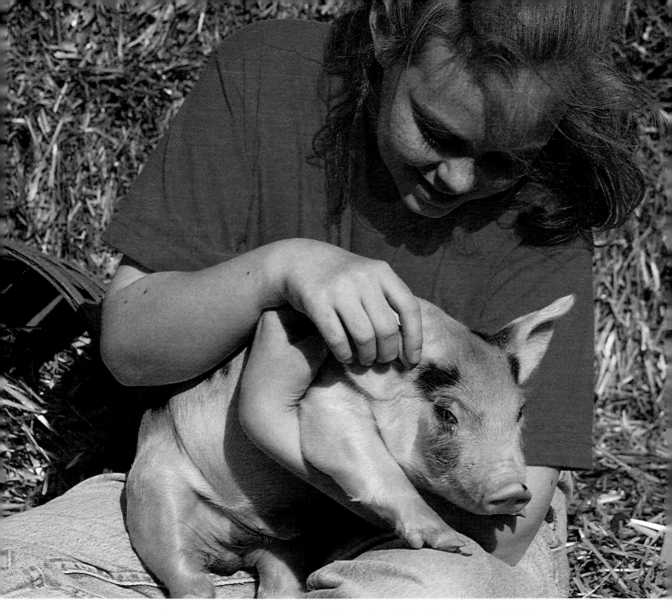

A girl's sense of touch tells her the piglet is dry and bristly

INSIDE THE HAND

A hand does what the brain tells it to. At the brain's signal, the hand moves through a series of 35 muscles. Fifteen of the muscles are in the lower arm. The other 20 are in the hand itself.

The muscles give hands and wrists strength and quickness. Baseball players have strong wrists that help control the swing of a bat.

The hands of a collector of poisonous snakes need to be quick, strong, and steady

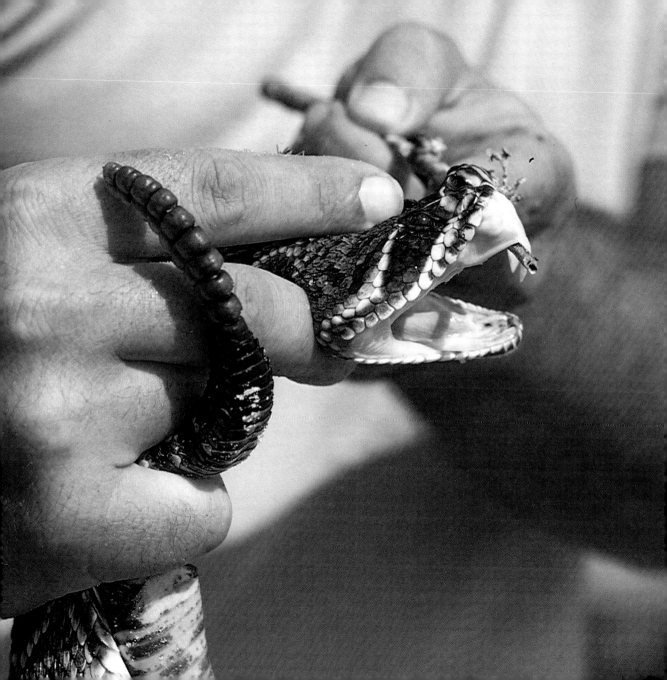

SENSE OF TOUCH

Leaves on a tree are sensitive to the slightest breeze. Our hands are sensitive to the lightest touch.

We have a sense of touch because of "feelers" in our skin. These feelers are called **nerves** (NERVZ). The hand is packed with nerves.

When the hand touches something, nerves take the message and send it to the brain. The brain then gives us the feeling, such as a light touch, heat, or cold.

The sense of touch in this girl's hand tells her this fish is wet and slimy

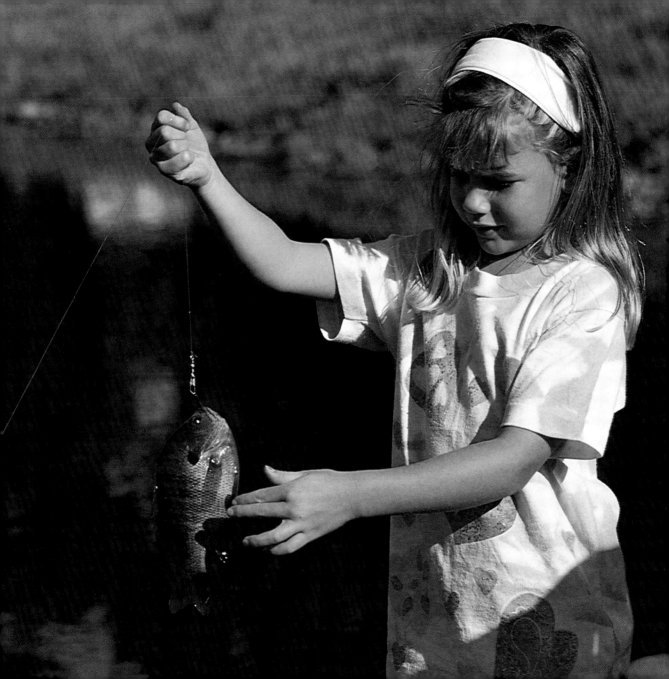

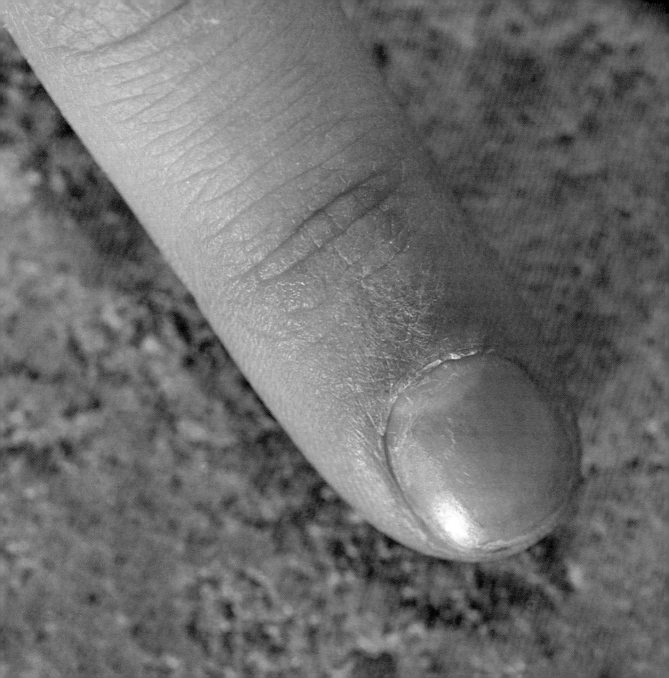

FINGERNAILS

The tips of fingers have small "nails." The nail is tough and fairly hard, so it helps protect fingertips.

If a nail is torn off, it will usually grow back. Nails continually grow, which is why we trim them.

Fingernails are made largely of a substance called **keratin** (KER et en). Keratin is the same material from which animal horns and hooves are made.

Human fingernails and toenails are made of keratin, the same material in cow hooves

HAND PROBLEMS

Because they are used so often, hands are often put at risk of injury. Broken or sprained fingers are common. A joint disease called arthritis can cripple hands.

Leaving fingers in cold air can cause frostbite. Frostbite occurs when the blood in the fingertips cannot keep the flesh warm. The flesh begins to freeze.

Frostbite can be prevented by keeping fingers in warm gloves or pockets.

The poisonous, bearded lizard of Mexico has a nasty bite, so a handler wisely protects a hand with a tough glove

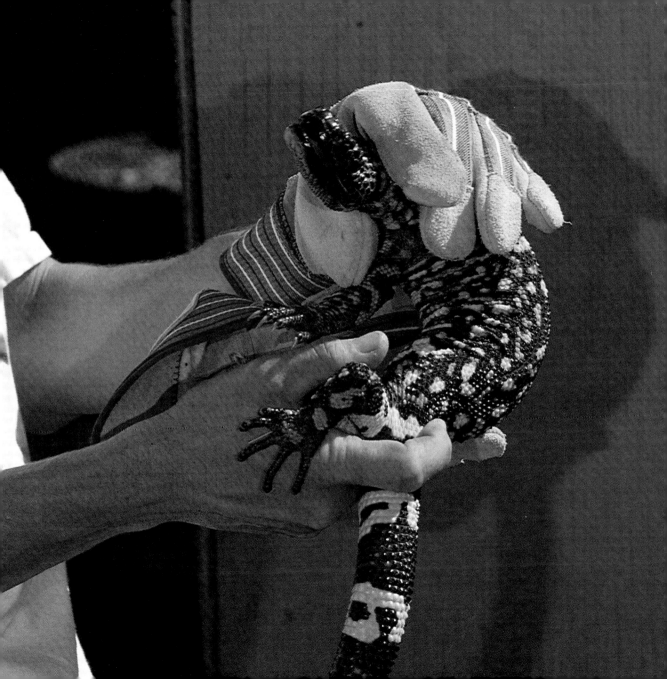

ANIMAL HANDS

We think of the word "hands" as being reserved for people. However, the "paws" of gorillas, chimpanzees, and orangutans could just as well be called hands. The hands of these apes look—and move—very much like our hands. An ape can scratch, grasp branches, and deliver food to its mouth with its hands.

Raccoons and bears use their front paws skillfully, but they lack the true fingers of apes and people.

Glossary

braille (BRAY el) — a system of writing using raised dots as letters so that blind people, by feeling the dots, can read

flexible (FLEHX uh bul) — able to bend easily and often

gesture (JEST yur) — a movement of the hand or body that carries a message

keratin (KER et en) — the hard material of which fingernails, horns, and hooves are made

nerves (NERVZ) — the sensitive "feelers" in the flesh that send messages to the brain

INDEX

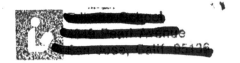